Haircentric

By Stephonia Roberts

Copyright ©

Haircentric
© 2015, Stephonia Roberts
Self publishing
mrsjacksbodyfood@hotmail.com

Introduction

I have been struggling with my hair for years because assumed notions that your hair defines who you are. I am always reminded of the biblical story of Samson and Delilah and his strength was in his hair. I would like for you to join me on my own personal journey as I look back to discover my own strengths, loving my hair, and acceptance of who I am.

It has been a long difficult road with enlightenment along the way by embracing myself and others.

This book is not about natural vs. relaxed or weaves but we are not our hair.

Acknowledgement

First of all I give thanks to The Almighty God for giving me so many gifts even when I do not use them properly He still stands by me, And Thanks go out to my husband Roland, and beautiful children Frank, Kristina, Cameron, Michaela, and Jara who trusts me more than I trust myself. I appreciate all those that have encouraged and inspired me over the years. And believed that I could do this thing especially Debbie for constantly encouraging me in all that I do.

To my sisters, DeLois (who recently passed away from pancreatic cancer), Ursula, and Sholonda I love you. And to my cousins Louise, Margie, Jennifer, Diane, Edie and Cassandra for their love and personal hair journey. A special shout out to my special daughters Stephanie, Samantha, Monique and Juanita!

For my cousin, Thelma (Tenchee) and Johnny Mae who first took care of my hair.

Special shout out to my friend since ninth grade, god mother of my first born. Girl, you are awesome Adrienne Jones-Johnson!

And most of all to my ace, ride or die, flee or fly bestie Jacqueline Aldridge Chatman you have seen me and saw right through me and found my heart!

Table of Contents

Chapter 1

My Journey

I recently received a book from a friend who happened to be a client about growing and loving your natural hair. I loved the book because it made me realize that I was not alone in my journey with issues of my own hair care regimen. My friend gave me the book after purchasing a few hair care items from me because she was amazed that all the years of trying to manage her natural hair that Mrs Jacks Natural & Organic Body Food products were the only ones that worked. Of course that made her curious to know why these products were different and it also made me feel fabulous giving me the confirmation that I was doing the right thing. She purchased the book, read it and passed it on to me. Cool friend huh?

Anyway, there were quite a few things in the book I was already familiar with especially, when it came to Western and Ayurvedic herbs for obtaining healthy hair. But, what had me was the author's journey from childhood to adulthood concerning the never ending issues with African American hair care, its growth, length, stigmatisms, the assembly line of hair care products, and the controversy of relaxed versus natural. It's all madness to me. I really related to the book very well deciding this was the journey that I needed to write about too. I used the title from a weekly blog that I was doing on social media about hair care called Haircentric.

Let's talk Haircentric; this is my word and my definition: a mix between the word hair and eccentric or other words crazy hair. Haircentric is about loving and growing my hair in relation to who I am and not how society thinks I should be! Dare to be different when it comes to your hair. Be Haircentric!!!!

I know there are many of us out there, women of African descent, women with coarse hair, curly hair or women that are just struggling to find their hair acceptable because they have been spoon fed to believe that they have bad hair. I grew up listening to that mess and straight hair was believed to be more acceptable because women with European ancestry had straight hair. This type of hair and beauty was considered angelic. Not only did Black women fall into that trap but, a large majority of Black men believed the same story which unknowingly helped to spread the propaganda of straight hair was better for African American women.

 When I was a young girl, I remember either having my hair braided or hot combed. If you had the patience for sitting at long periods of time for braiding it wasn't so bad unless you had a cousin like mine that could braid to the scalp so tight that your ethnicity changed from African American to African Chinese. Then, there would be the little bumps that sometimes would appear around your hairline especially by your ears and maybe the nape of your neck. Of course there are the sleepless nights from hair so tight that you would have a headache. To this day I cannot have anything on my head at night; I go crazy and refuse to sleep with rollers in my hair. I definitely do not wrap my hair at night because I flip out if I feel the slightest tension on my scalp. So, what is a girl to do?

Now, there were times that I rather have my hair straightened with a pressing comb because once my hair was trained it would stay straight for several weeks. One day when my mom was pressing my hair she accidently dropped the hot comb. The handle had become too hot and greasy. The hot comb popped off my forehead to only run down the side of my face to give me a new burn mark which, my mom immediately put butter on (so my cheek could cook some more) . And all this to have straight hair!

For the most part I was a tomboy and I would sweat my hair out before the next day. My hair would be filled with grass and leaves from playing side line kill football. I was not a prissy girl but, I did want my hair to be nice and if this is what I would have to do to obtain it! And with a sigh, okay!

I remember when I first dyed my hair I was 15. I was fascinated by the color of auburn because when I was around ten I found my birth certificate. I remember on the birth certificate my hair color at birth was auburn. I felt special to have red hair and to this day I love red heads regardless of race I just get all goo goo ga ga over red heads. The only problem after my hair was dyed my mom decided to give me a pointed shaped afro. I was a sophomore in high school with a hair style of a carrot. All I needed was a green top. That same year I received a green toboggan, scarf and mittens for Christmas. I looked like a hot mess.

I did enjoy the color but, that pointed hair doo like a fuzzy Dan Akroyd in the 1993 Coneheads movie was not such a thrilling part of my life. I had to deal with the shape and the dryness of my hair as well. I kept a drawer full of old school hair care products like Royal Crown, Sulfur 8, and some Afro Sheen to help manage my hair.

I was still relaxer free at that time because I thought getting a relaxer was for rich folks so I wasn't in that status yet, but a relaxer was something that I secretly desired. I had a mom and grandmother that came from the old school so pressing, plaiting, and braiding were the options for managing your hair. There were a few other hairstyles that I wore like the page boy when it was pressed, the wavy hair which was just water with hair grease brushed real well. Every now and then if I wanted it really curly I would just twist my hair up and roll it using torn paper sack. Let me know if you are relating!

My mom, acquired a new job with longer hours, better wages and she didn't have time to do my hair anymore plus I was older but, I appreciated that my mom would send me to the barber shop, *The Chopping Block*, every two weeks to get my hair done. The owner of the shop was a middle aged man that had an eye for cutting and grooming hair. Every now and then he would attend to my hair and finally passed me on to one of the ladies that he had hired who would wash, press and curl my hair. I was now becoming prissy. I grew up with the idea that this is what you needed to do to look pretty and have nice hair. Then something wonderful happened in the late 70's. The hair care market for Blacks exploded like a riot. Jeri Curl came onto the scene like an Afro Sheen. (I hoped you enjoyed the pun). My mom let me get a Jeri curl around the age of 18 and as we say it was on and popping (especially that juice running down your neck)!

I suffered for a while with the greasy pillow, greasy shirt collar and the sweaty hair bag until I married moving overseas with my military husband. There weren't too many hair products available at the commissary and not many local beauticians were familiar with Black hair care. I kept the Jeri Curl for awhile until I had my son and by that time my hair got so big they called the hair style a *Cake*. I recall though going to a beauty shop on one of the nearby military bases in my area getting my hair done by a Caucasian lady who appeared to be pretty intrigued with my hair. I look back now because it made me laugh because my hair was just as foreign to her as it was foreign to me. It was also strange for me to allow her to do my hair because I was wondering what she thought of the texture and the feel of it. In the past it was normal for Black women to groom white women hair. So this was a little awkward to me. For a few years I managed my hair the best that I could. I think that's what began my journey with relaxers not knowing that I had already used chemicals such as perms beginning with the Jeri Curl. Silly, I did not find out to decades later that a perm and a relaxer were two different things. Of course it was a few decades after that before I realized the dangers of chemically processing your hair.

As, I stumbled in and out of hair styles and trying to find an identity for my hair I had enlisted in the Navy where it was the first time that I had gotten a Caucasian perm. You heard me a perm not a relaxer. I went to the beauty shop on base and of course there was no one that looked liked me once again to do my hair. I allowed the beautician to put on an Ogilvie, giving my hair a curlier texture when it was done. So, I looked like I still had a Jeri curl. Whew, the hair saga continued. It was manageable and I didn't have to do too much to it. I could get in the water not worrying about getting my hair wet. I could go to bed at night not having to sleep with my head in awkward positions. I wouldn't mess up my hair and I felt as if I could be normal.

Don't get me wrong I have met many beautiful Black women with gorgeous hair natural or processed. But, I know we all have had two things in common: not getting your hair wet and don't run your fingers through my hair. Matter of fact when I had finally completed my transition from a relaxed state to an afro one of the first person that approached me was a Caucasian gentleman. I was friends with him and before I knew it he had his hand in the middle of my hair! He was reminiscing from days of old and I had to snap him out of his *Get Christi Love* scenario before I actually snapped off his fingers.

Some Black women have what we call "good hair", those are the ones that their hair was more manageable not so coarse nor curly, easy to run a comb and brush through. They didn't have to flat iron their hair because it was already straight due to less strands that bind a follicle together. (That was my scientific approach). When you saw that type of hair you would say, "Oh she has a good grade of hair," This was like your hair was getting a D or an F for a grade. There were many women in my youth that had that Grade A hair and my grandmother was one of those ladies. For the most part she usually kept her hair in plaits and occasionally a bun or two. I think her major concern in life with her hair as she aged was becoming gray. We had a lot of Grecian Formula 16 around the house that was as close to chemical processing and dying her hair I would see. Much later years, she gave up dying her hair and begun wearing a wig. Her hair was silky gray. I really never knew why, she didn't have thinning hair because she wore that wig like a skull cap. And to think about it was never on her head straight either. During the early 70's natural hair was not an issue because we were still preoccupied with a good old fashioned straightening comb.

Another Grade A hair person was my Aunt Lola who had the prettiest salt and pepper hair that reached to her shoulders when she wore it down. But, for most of her life time it was always plaited in two plaits coiled up into a bun. I remember asking her once about how she kept it so beautiful and she told me she gave it a 100 brush strokes. This must have been a passed down truth because my grandma did the same thing as well. I really don't know how true the 100 brush strokes are but, I know it gave you the opportunity to be still and be quite. It may have some spiritual connotations as well along with some physical attributes like building up your biceps too. I was definitely being funny in this sentence.

My mom, who was an Afrocentric goddess, wore an afro for years. The nape of her neck was caressed with baby fine tendrils. This is known to some of us as the kitchen. I can't explain that one but just keep along with me. She was like Cleopatra Jones tall, sexy and beautiful. That was my image of a strong Black woman which is still the epitome of a woman to me. I believe the time frame of the 70's set the stage with free love, flower children, and civil rights leading the Black is Beautiful movement. The image of a held high fisted Black woman with an afro is embedded subconsciously in our minds as a symbol of power while earlier decades offered the Black mother with scarf tied on her head, an apron around her body, and house shoes on set examples of a happy loving servant. Cooking, cleaning and managing her household along with her employer's home became her attributes for the time. It was stereotypical of the times because many women I grew up around in my hometown wore that attire and job. The afro seemed to symbolize freedom and beauty which became very common because it was cool.

My mom had a picture of her when she was twenty-eight years old. She had an afro that was beautiful and I would stare at it in awe. A few years ago we went out to a Christmas event where we took pictures. I noticed the beauty in my own afro and how much I looked like my mom back in the day. I put the picture we had taken next to the picture that my mom had back then. I thought not only did I look like my mom the same way she looked in that picture but I also realized that I too was a strong Black woman. I had finally embraced my ethnicity and was happy!

Well, we know now with the progression of technology everything else has to move forward as well as Black hair care. There are more hair alternatives from wigs, weave, extensions, and sew-ins. I know over time I have tried them all looking for the right hairstyle and process. Once, I had my first daughter I knew I wouldn't have to do too much to take care of her she was a Grade A too but, how did that happen? Could it be it was in one of her parents DNA? Her daddy folks had thick hair and so did my folks so what happened? These are the things unfortunately we care about. I always told people that I was skipped over a generation with my hair. I use to say the same thing about the boys in our family with their hazel eyes. I would say that the girls were regular with muddy brown eyes but, that too I had to learn to change my mind set.

My oldest daughter, Kristina had soft gentle twisting curls that I could easily brush out and part into many sections. I could add those pretty little colored barrettes too. She was a little tender headed but her hair was easily combed. No relaxers for her but, little did I know that my child was getting caught up in black hair stereotypes. How her hair should be according to main stream society. I remember she begged and begged me when she was around ten to get her hair relaxed and of course I said no because I knew she didn't need it. She didn't have to go through the mental and physical anguish that I had endured with my hair type, curling, pressing, hot combing, relaxing and so no to Kristina no!

But, you know when you have a persistent child that wears you down and within the next two years she was twelve I finally gave in. Off to the beauty shop we went. I allowed her to have her hair relaxed. We purchased one made just for little girls' hair. It didn't take long to relax her hair. It was beautiful and I left the beauty shop with a satisfied child. Her first beauty shop hair style was a French roll and during that time we lived in an apartment complex with a swimming pool. She loved to go swimming and it only took a few weeks to realize my daughter was losing her hair from the chlorine in the pool. It was summer and I could hardly keep her out. My child who had beautiful hair that I could twist down to her shoulders now, had hair that barely came to the nape of her neck. The so called Grade A was still there weaker and the length had gone. Now, after sixteen years she still has trouble growing her hair.

When, she was old enough to manage her own hair she became interested in Quick weave. I continued to watch my daughter's once beautiful hair mutate into mainstream hair fashion, continually adding tracks, suffocating hair follicles and removing glue that would be on the walls of the bathroom shower or stuck on towels. We lost many towels to hair glue.

A few years ago we finally convinced her to at least get her dead ends trimmed which to my surprise she visited a beautician at Wally World and came home with a complete bob. All of her hair had been chopped off and what were left were beautiful ringlets all over her head. Her head was beautiful and that style looked perfect on her. The bob made her appear taller, slimmer and she looked very natural in it. That only lasted two weeks at the most before she added more weave into her hair and now it came to her shoulder in some awful Cleopatra style.

I still cringe thinking about that particular hair style. But, once again I had to understand it was her hair and her journey. I was still dealing with my own.

About a decade ago I became part of the *Assembly Line* where I went regularly to get my hair done. It was horrible. I would take off the whole day from work paid or unpaid having a 10 o'clock am appointment only to leave at midnight sometimes. Seriously, my beautician was great in doing my hair because it was short then. She was good at what she did but, she constantly overbooked her customers and then she would let her family come in bumping your appointment. Especially, if they claimed that had some important function to attend that day so, I got tired of it. I got smart thinking Saturday appointments would be better. I would be in the parking lot of the business for a 730am appointment only to realize that several other patrons sitting in their cars. They were waiting for the same time slot! And to make matters worse she wouldn't show up to an hour later. Those moments caused a lot of frustration but once you had your hair done she had you looking beautiful. You felt like a new person with that fresh hair doo.

I remember one Saturday morning it was me with four other ladies parked in the parking lot. I was the first to arrive and when I saw the other cars I became annoyed praying that their appointments were later than mine. I wanted to be the first in the door. After, thirty minutes of waiting the beautician showed up. All the ladies got out of their cars except for one lady. She was asleep and no one bothered to wake her. Of course I was still waiting to be seen when the lady came into the shop cursing obscenities to everyone that was there. I felt bad for her but; she did take a good nap. We were no further along than she was once some of the beautician family members came along. My beautician would have one cousin wash your hair, one put on the relaxer, one put you under the drier but, for some strange reason those same family members would be finished getting their hair done before you could get your hair curled. Your 7:30am appointment actually turned into a 04:00pm appointment and your whole day would be gone. I would lose vacation day, $70 or $80 bucks for the doo, a day to run and do other things. It took me a while before I finally realized it wasn't worth it! I needed to look around for a beautician that had my time in mind.

My next Haircentric adventure was adding weave to my hair. I found another beautician that was good at weaving and I didn't have to stay long to get my hair done but, eventually there was a problem. I developed two bald spots on each side of my temples that ran about the length of my index finger. You could not mistake the absence of hair follicles due to the track glue. I was horrified as it was another blow to my hair journey. Weave made me more attractive filling in the places where my hair wasn't full, or just having a professional kept look but it became a bad thing. It caused your hair to become brittle, split ends and created hair loss. Even after knowing that like I an addict I would still dabbled in it from time to time. I made excuses because it was a quick fix and like a hair addict I would tell myself weave wasn't as prominent in my life and I could change if I wanted. As I tried to kick the quick weave habit I would see many Black women with these wonderful plastic like hairstyle reminding me of Barbie or Chrissy dolls. They had hair that would keep as long as you kept it. I was depressed.

My next hair journey I heard about Sew-In thinking it was a wonderful idea much better than weave. I felt my best with manageable hair with bounce and length but, I'm not great with sitting long enough to get my hair braided. I realized I had to find a happy medium and the sew-in did not take as long as I thought. It made me feel beautiful and I have to admit till this day I still like it. And another thing I noticed that I didn't do that pat-a-tat-tat as much!

The familiar sometimes spontaneous patting that you see women doing to stop their hair from itching was curious at best. These involuntary compulsions raised eyebrows and questions to the strange behavior. . But of course we know not that the scalp wasn't receiving good circulation and air. The hair was literally being suffocated. While, we may not think nothing of it now it will come to bite us in our older years. Our body slows down reducing the amount of nutrients and supplements that were required in our youth for the necessary energy. Wear and tear and improper diet along with increased inflammation begins to bombard our bodies. As we age our body's changes due to lack of hormones producing drier skin, loss of bone density, rashes and creating dry brittle hair. Hair loss or thinning hair is seen quite a lot in my profession especially Alopecia. It has become a task to make women understand the dangers of chemicals on their hair along with hysterectomies as well. I believe that they go hand in hand because you lose a lot of hormones once you remove your womb. How many older women in their sixties and beyond have you seen that grew up with the relaxers and wigs, and have had hysterectomies? Some of them are now practically bald and suffering from other ailments. Now, mind you not all women are like that but there is a pattern. My mother who never had a relaxer still has a head full of hair but is starting to thin in her 70's because she loves to cut her hair which may cause it to stop growing. Also, she never had a full hysterectomy. I know for most women who have had a hysterectomy hair loss is natural and only lasts for a few weeks to a few months but, that is not the case if you already had other underlying health issues that cause hair to become weak and brittle such as perms and relaxers.

Another type of hair loss can be caused by medication. For example I once was taking a prescription drug that I had to take six times a day that stated clearly that for African Americans one of the sides of effects of the medicine was hair loss. I was on the medicine for a year and it was daunting every time I would comb or wash my hair. I would lose enough hair to add on the head of a Chrissy doll (Chrissy dolls came out in the 70's and you could pull her hair in the middle of her head and it would grow longer). And at the time, I had a relaxer making the decision to go ahead chopping my hair to get that entire chemical out. Unfortunately, it was a health decision that caused me to look at my hair differently instead of it being some awe knowing inspiring cultural thing.

Whatever the decision I'm glad I had the gumption to do so. And while I was learning to deal with my own head I had already made a conscious decision for my youngest daughter to keep from adding chemicals to her hair. Wow, that baby was born with beautiful hair and had *that chic curly I want to style and wear my wig hair if only it would grow like that type of hair.* For years I would struggle to tame it but looking back I really do not know why that was so important then. She had beautiful curly locks. I actually have an old wig stored somewhere in a drawer that is just like her hair type that reminding how beautiful my daughter's hair was at that time. It's crazy now thinking how I went out buying that wig for myself but I was trying to abolish my child's natural curls. That was just dumb! Her hair was so beautiful, thick and curly that I would spend hours before school trying to put her hair in pony tails, twisted pony tails, and little plaits so she could have the perfect farmer's square patch markings in her head like if someone flying overhead was going to mistake her head for prime farming land. As, I begin to lose the struggle I let me older daughter deal with trying to comb her hair really not knowing how to deal with hair that was naturally curly and beautiful it seemed we were losing the battle, with tender head, wrong combs, ineffective detangler shampoos, lack of acceptance and then there were the days I just didn't want to tackle her hair. I am ashamed to say that there were times her hair was so matted that we had to cut mounds of her hair out. We were too busy trying to brush her hair straight. Finally, one morning while getting ready for church I had to do her hair, it took me two hours to get it in the popular little kid hairstyle with the little barrettes. I was so annoyed that I remember being at church upset and my older daughter was concerned wanting to fix the problem. So we agreed for a change and bought a *Just for Me* relaxer and while I was at work the next day I received a picture on my cell. They had completed my baby girl's hair. It was beautiful flowing down her back. I never knew that her hair was that long and now, I would enjoy styling my daughter's hair not worrying about her tenderness. But, boy was I wrong because six months later my daughter had lost the majority of her length! Her hair was barely in a pony tail and all those luscious curls that were natural had been processed out and obliterated.

I was horrified what I had done to my daughter's hair due to a lack of knowledge and self worth. Even though I had fought so hard with my oldest daughter about getting a relaxer I just gave up and through my hands up. And now with my youngest daughter does hair I agreed out of frustration no longer wanting to deal with struggling to groom her hair. She had the top of the list for Grade A curly hair and suddenly you find yourself going to the beauty supply asking for Coarse Yaki hair to get that beautiful natural care free look.

After several attempts of trying to correct the damaged done to her hair, a few more relaxers that stated were made just for children I realized that there was only one way coming from this hair debacle. I needed to cut the relaxer out to let her hair grow back free of chemicals. My youngest has been relaxer free longer than I have. It's been almost five years for her and now she has length and thickness. We didn't get the entire wonderful S curl pattern back but we get to see it when she washes her hair. Her hair is soft and manageable.

Ironically as I write this story she does have a sew-in because she wanted to have her hair braided while she played basketball. She washes and conditions her hair often and I am happy to say that she uses my homemade shampoos and conditioners as well. I am thankful that she is young accepting it's okay to have natural hair and hopefully this experience will stick with her while she learns loving herself as well as her hair.

Now, I know most men don't stress out about their hair like women do because it doesn't take as much time to groom. I remember putting a texturizer on one of my male cousin when we were young. I remember putting his head under the kitchen sink faucet running water to rinse the lye out of his hair and as he was saying ouch I could see the burn marks on his scalp. He had sores on his head that lasted for weeks. I think that summer I must have put on several relaxers and texturizer on a few other male cousins as well. Everyone was using the Afro Sheen products and S curl to get that look. For the boys that look was crazy so enough on that subject until I had my first born son Frank.

As a baby Frank had beautiful hair like most babies. We took care of his hair with the normal grooming processes of brushing, combing and washing and it grew well too. His dad always kept him clean cut and he had nice little curls. I really don't remember too many issues with my son's hair but, when he was promoted to the ninth grade his hair doo and type did a major overhaul. He asked me to put a texturizer *The Duke* on his head and wham he had the *Billy D Williams* hair doo. The girls went wild especially with the little ringlets that formed a frame around his face like fringes off an old jacquard curtain. He was the man and he kept his hair pretty much oiled up. He was definitely handsome. I guess after the fad wore off so did his hairstyle as he went back to natural. I saw him a few times with braids but most of time that clean barber shop fade did the trick. My youngest son when he was born had sandy straight hair which as a toddler turned into big nice curls. My stepfather use to tell me that my son had the Lyle Lovett hairstyle. Lyle Lovett is an American country singer, writer and actor with big hair and my baby boy had this one big curl on his forehead that demanded attention giving him the Lyle Lovett look. When it was time for his first real hair cut his father suggested that we take him to a major hair cutting chain. We were greeted by a friendly host and assigned a beautician/barber. Once my son was in the chair the young woman that was assigned to cut his hair seemed confused and overwhelmed with the task that lay before her. She wasn't accustomed to cutting biracial hair but until his dad spoke with her she calmed down managing to do pretty well. I do recall feeling a little bit discouraged and frustrated. Perhaps she felt that his hair was too coarse or curly for her to cut but that's just letting me give her an excuse it was exactly what I thought it was and that was just plain old stupidity and cultural ignorance on her part.

Sometimes, we prejudge a thing due to stereotypes and we lose sight of a great opportunity to learn more. I never really had a problem of different races working on my hair. I thought beauticians were taught to be universal when it came to hair types. For example, the beauty school I attended to get my hair done was co-ed, black and white. They would eventually have the experience in becoming a great barber or beautician knowing how to do all hair types.

Next child to talk about is my middle daughter who has beautiful hair also but her ancestry is African American and Caucasian. When she was little she had very long Farah Faucet type hair. It would tangle or rat up just like any other hair but, a brush was better than a comb. It was easy to manage once it was detangled and I was able to create those wonderful piggy tails that I had been striving. Her hair was beautiful, thick and was my glory until one day I noticed that she too was having issues with her beautiful locks.

She didn't like her curls anymore. She said that when she took a shower her hair would curl and frizz up really bad and she wanted her hair straighter. So, I bought the best flat irons around and watched her spend hours flat ironing her hair. She had thickness and length which made it tedious to reach that straight hair look. I searched high and low for a beautician that could tame her hair and we ended up at a Mexican beauty salon that was familiar with her hair type. They did very well in giving her those looks that she so much wanted but that didn't last for long. She also went through the phase of wanting weave. Yes, weave but she also did micro braids and some extensions previously. She kept up with straight hair from the ninth to the eleventh grade but, then her senior year I noticed a light had been turned on for her as well. Even though her hair grade did not require relaxers or perms she longed for the natural look and put away the flat iron for awhile embracing her natural curl pattern. I asked her once why did she do it and she proudly said that she wanted to be free to enjoy her natural hair. I am very proud of her and some may say well that's easy for her to do since she has that so called Grade A and she's mixed but, it's the subliminal message that straight hair is the way to go is not always accurate.

Back to me for a minute, I remember one of the sexiest hairstyles I had was done at a barber college. I didn't have to wait long and I was given a relaxer, no weaves, and no extensions, my hair was rolled up in big rollers. And my attendant was a wonderful Asian woman who gave me a *sister girl curl (at least that what she called it).* My hair was long with Shirley Temple like curls. I enjoyed the freedom that I felt with curls holding without the hard gels, stiff mousse or spritz.

I never liked too much junk on my head to hold a style, it either got sprayed in my eyes, the fumes were harsh to breath in, and I just didn't like that frozen in time hair doo.

I wanted my hair to have movement which this particular hair style did just that. A few times I went back to the barber college just to get wraps until finances kept me from my hair ritual. That's the other issue I want to talk about: the money that is involved in keeping up your hair. If you don't have the money to do your hair then what happens to your hair? You should learn to take care of it without the hassle of costly products, expensive stylists, and long waiting lines at the beauty shop. What you are gaining is valuable time spent on your on head learning more about how to take care of your own hair. I use to laugh when I would go to a beauty shop. I would see beauticians working feverishly on someone else's head and their own hair looked like a mess. The conclusion I drew was they were so busy trying to make ladies heads cute that they didn't have time for themselves or the other option was they had no clue about hair. I did occasionally run into the clueless stylist and heaven forbid you were lucky if you got out with your hair still attached to your scalp.

When I was in my late twenties I had a hair style called a Freeze. It was rolled up to the nape of my neck. Boy, I thought I was something special with that hair style. After several times of wearing that hair style I noticed that my head would itch in two spots. When I would scratch I noticed that my scalp felt different. I washed my hair finding that I had two bald spots one on each side of my head like horns. I was concerned and made a doctor's appointment. The doctor told me it could be stress that created the hair loss. No, the stress was created from the loss of my hair. No more Freeze hair styles after that but, you think I would have learned by then. Having issues with your hair is like having children. You forget about the pain you incurred with each child but, you have another. I dealt with different hairstyles and before I knew it 15 years had passed. I was really heavy into the Quick weave adoring how the hair would drape my face and you can obtain almost any hair style you wanted. I wore the weave for a while because it was easy and fast but, one of those days when I was taking the weave out I noticed that at the temple of my hairline down to my ears that I was missing hair. The weird thing about it the bald spot was in the shape of the track where the hair was attached with that awful glue. I jumped in the shower to get the rest of the weave out of my hair and leaned against the shower wall and cried. It seemed like this was too big a price to pay to have nice hair styles.

I wanted to be a free was a wash and wear type of girl. I didn't want to just dangle my feet at the edge of the swimming pool and not jump in because I was afraid of getting my hair wet. I wanted to spend a Saturday morning with my family instead of getting up early like I was going to work coming out of the beauty shop a whole day later. I wanted to sleep comfortably on a pillow not concerned if my $70.00 hair doo got messed up during the middle of the night. I just wanted to be free and then came the wigs. I had so many wigs at one time that I had short, long, straight or curly. All I had to do was brush my hair back and put on a stocking cap which after a while would have my head hurting. Sometimes the combs that were attached to the interior of the wig would begin to stab my scalp after awhile. Wigs, Wigs, and Wigs, I had had enough of those too. So, what is a girl to do? Don't get me wrong if you like relaxer then that's your thing then so it is. I was telling someone the other day I wonder what cultural groups spends the most money on hair care products? Even though I may not know the correct answer I do know that research shows that Black women spend more than a trillion dollars on hair care products yearly on weave. That's a lot and it's because of two reasons, we want to look our best and it's the social psychosis of how beauty is defined when it comes to hair.

Honestly, if it wasn't for the affliction that occurred in my life there's a possibility I would still relax my hair. And, I will say that I am greatful for it because it has brought me a sense of freedom. My new old hairstyle wasn't initially accepted by my husband because he too was part of the myth. I had to educate him for both our sakes realizing that some Black men propagated the propaganda as well about Black women hair care and regimen.

I am one of those women that really like short hair but for years I had to make a choice not to cut my hair because my husband's disapproval.

His statement was, "if I wanted a wife with short hair I would have married a boy". Well, after a few times of refusing to dress my hair properly he realized it was costly, frustrating, and took too much of our Saturdays away. He eventually acquiescence but, by that time I was really enjoying my natural afro and felt like I was a pro. Later, I made the big chop leaving enough hair to look like a small afro bob. I embraced the first months with small baby steps then as it began to grow it took shape and had a life force of its own. I noticed that I would dress according to my afro. I loved the change it brought in me. I felt Angela Davis and Pam Greer all in one. I felt empowered which I hadn't felt that way in a long time. I walked with a confidence of having natural beauty despite the odds that were brought on by peer pressure and society. I was a Beautiful Black butterfly ready to spread my wings and pollinate the world on being a Natural woman. I even found a few hair picks actually wearing one in the back of my head for awhile to see if anyone would notice. I felt attractive and I felt me again. I brought an array of silk flowers to adorn my hair and occasionally I would actually wear a live flower only if I could keep the bees from following me around.

When I would go out I would always have other Black women approach me telling me how they liked my afro and share their fears of going natural. I would even have a few folks that would asked to touch it bringing don't you put your hand in a black woman's head to another whole level. For example, a friend who perhaps had a 70's flash back saw me with my new doo and of course I did think my afro made me sexy. In a flash before I knew it he had his hand deep inside my afro rocking my head back and forth exclaiming all the while how much he loved my afro. I was annoyed but, I let him have his momentary relapse and sucked in the complement. I never received that many compliments before with my relaxed hairstyles. The attention was about how much did that cost, and is that your real hair or you would have fingers feeling for tracks in your head.

Whatever you choice make sure that you take care of your hair because it's definitely an extension of who you are. Remember the story of Samson who had beautiful hair and that is where he drew his strength but, most importantly invest in knowing what the best products for you and your hair. As Dr Phoenix Austin says in her book and the title, "If *You Love It, it will Grow.* "

C hapter 2 Knowing Your Hair History

Hair has been established in three main types depending on ethnic group which are Afro-Caribbean, Asian, and Caucasian with Asian hair being the dominant of all hair types. So this brings up a great point. Asian hair is usually smaller in thickness than the other types but it grows faster than the rest of the other ethnic hair types. Thus, because of the thickness it appears to be full and it has been found to react better to hair care products than its counterparts especially hair loss products. It is also stronger than other types, more able to recuperate from damages, and has the longest hair growth cycle of nine years which makes it the ideal hair for extensions. And the largest of the Asian producers is the Indian market which plays an extremely vital role in weave and hair extensions. It is said that Indian hair is considered the best in the market for its quality and length. Indian women from the villages don't use any chemicals, take great care of their hair, and comb it frequently using only coconut oil . The Indian hair weave business began around the 1980s for producing wigs, but the real boom took place during the last 10 years with the increased popularity of hair extensions. Even though the market in the African American community is notoriously known for the largest demand of weave due to the diminishing of Afros in the 60's and 70's which gave way to chemical relaxers and extensions. Weaves have been controversial within the African American community, as they have been viewed as conforming to a European standard of beauty. I personally have heard this so many times that I became confused because of that myth. I decided to research the origins of weave and found that extensions, weaves, and wigs have been around since the ancient of days specifically in Egypt around 3400 BC. Hair extensions were considered fashionable status quo and it remained symbolic throughout the Georgian, Romantic, Victorian and Edwardian eras. These elaborate creations began the styles of the French wigs, Apollo knot styles, the pompadour, and even the 60's beehive hairstyle to obtain a sophisticated appeal.

Even though it was much of a rave in European countries weaves and extensions still have its origins from Africa. In Africa, many tribes were identified by their hairstyles thus creating elaborate braided designs to identify, beautify and give social recognition. Then slavery entered the scene and slavers may have known this or just thought the hair styles were ugly or nasty but, they begin immediately cutting the hair of those that have been captured stripping their identity and culture away. Once colonized throughout America and Europe female slaves began wearing scarves or rags to adorn their head out of necessity to protect the hair from the effects of hard labor, harshness of the sun, and dustiness of working in the fields. It definitely was not a fashion statement. There was no time for special hair grooming without negative consequences from the slave owner. It is still popular in Africa and conscious African American women to wear scarves known as wraps as head dressings for adornments.

Once slavery was abolished the adaptation of being in a different land was difficult for those who wanted to maintain hair with natural oils of their homeland. Adapting was the main approach bringing the desired ideal prized Anglo women hairstyles to the forefront for Black women. Achieving straight hair became the norm for a people that had been emotionally and physically stripped of their culture learning to slowly adapt to a whole new life of hardship. And still the ideology of straight hair has a hold on the African American community but with more choosing the route of natural hair that mindset is slowly changing. Now if we can get a better understanding of organic versus chemically processed products we can establish new rules of hair care products in all cultural outlets.

When, I began writing I wanted to include all hair cultures because we spend so much wasted time over our differences we forget sometimes to look at the commonality. We all have hair growing on our heads or somewhere on our bodies. We all have been subjugated to stereotypes. I wanted to take away some of those myths. Over the last decade I have seen all hair type crossing over due to new products, versatile hairstyles, and racial diversity. Hair can be used as a medium for consideration as artistic expression. The interchangeable hairstyles, shows, and modeling have propelled hair doos into the limelight giving stylists the opportunity to show the best in coiffeurs. Knowing your hair type is extremely important and its condition. Knowing how your body works can be found in your hair. It is important to know your hair type and condition. This brings me to how our hair retains moisture in three forms; normal, dry or oily hair. How it grows can either be straight, coarse, wavy, curly or kinky. And then there are sub issues such as problematic hair like dandruff, alopecia, eczema or thinning hair.

And since, I am no expert but can only talk about my own hair and those of my family members which range from all the mentioned above.

Below are brief definitions of the three hair types:

Normal hair is defined as healthy hair it's neither dry nor oily. It looks great and has a nice luster to it. The only time that normal hair changes are because of health related issues and poor diet.

Dry hair is just like it is dry hair that becomes brittle, fly away, damaged, tangled and broken. This usually happens when the sebaceous glands are not making enough sebum to lubricate the follicles of your hair. A lot of times we worsen the condition with the chlorine in swimming pools, salt water from the beach, over exposure to the sun and most importantly to much tinting and coloring of the hair. Hair gels are not your friend. I have dry hair and that has not always been the case but because of meds and illnesses my hair has taking a different course. A lot of kinky hair falls into this category.

Oily hair is when your sebaceous glands produce too much sebum and therefore you have an excess amount of oil in your hair. Eventually weighing the hair down, making it to heavy to hold a curl and becomes lanky. Oily hair is a sign of ill health and one thing more we tend to wash the hair frequently to remove the oiliness thus more oil is produce. But, if you go around with oily hair you look nasty so what are you to do? Many bone straight hair types fall into this category.

Now that we got the types out of the way let's go to the next chapter to define classification and texture.

Chapter 3 Hair Grading System

There are two types of systems that are used to classify our hair, one being Andre Walker's Hair Type Classification System which is more effective and will use as the example. This chart below is the most commonly used chart to help determine hair types. Here is a breakdown of the hair types along with how each curls appears:

Type	Hair Texture	Hair Description
1a	Straight (Fine/Thin)	Very Soft, Shiny, Hard to hold a curl, hair tends to be oily, hard to damage.
1b	Straight (Medium)	Has lots of body. (i.e. more volume, more full)
1c	Straight (Coarse)	Hard to curl (i.e. bone straight). Most East Asians fall into this category.
2a	Wavy (Fine/Thin)	Can accomplish various styles. Definite "S" pattern. Hair sticks close to the head. Fine, thin and very easy to handle; easily straightened or curled
2b	Wavy (Medium)	A bit resistant to styling. Hair tends to be frizzy. Medium-textured z
2c	Wavy (Coarse)	Hair has thicker waves. Also resistant to styling. Hair tends to be frizzy.
3a	Curly (Loose	Thick & full with lots of body. Definite "S" pattern.

	Curls)	Hair tends to be frizzy. Can have a combination texture. Curls are naturally big, loose and usually very shiny. Circumference: sidewalk-chalk size
3b	Curly (Tight Curls)	Medium amount of curl. Can have a combination texture. Bouncy ringlets to tight corkscrews. Circumference: Sharpie size
3c	Curly (Corkscrews)	Tight curls in corkscrews. The curls can be either kinky, or very tightly curled, with lots and lots of strands densely packed together. Getting this type of hair to blow dry straight is more challenging than for 3a or 3b, but it usually can be done The very tight curls are usually fine in texture
4a	Kinky (Soft)	Tightly coiled. Very Fragile. Has a more defined curly pattern when stretched, has an "S" pattern, much like curly hair. It tends to have more moisture than 4b; has a definite curl pattern
4b	Kinky (Wiry)	Tightly coiled. Very Fragile. Less defined curly pattern. Has more of a "Z" shaped pattern. The hair bends in sharp angles like the letter "Z"; has a cotton-like feel. Does not retain water well. Shrinks up to 75% actual length. Susceptible to hair breakage, dryness, and damage

Finding your correct hair pattern and type can become very helpful in understanding how your hair grows.

Weave & Extension Grading System

I always was interested in weaves and tracks especially when I would go to the beauty supply stores noticing that each hair package would have numbers on it. I guess it was a system to help you know what type of hair you were purchasing versus Yaki, curly or Remy. So I wanted to know more.

I researched the information and found some interesting factors. There might be some validity to the system but, it all began as a marketing ploy for hair weave companies. As consumers we help to perpetuate this system idea. Supposedly, the higher the letter rating is the better the quality of hair. In my findings there have been several upgrades with 3A which in recent years was top of the line and then another upgrade reappeared perhaps by another company trying to out weave the best of the 3 A's company by creating a 6A. And then wow there is a 10A which I want go into that but try to stick to the basic theory.

There is no governing body that regulates these ratings, nor is there a standard set of requirements that need to be met in order to give your hair a certain rating.

Some sources say 3A means it is all virgin hair, 5A guarantees the cuticles are in the same direction. In fact well established, reputable companies don't even bother with this nonsense. A rating system is only helpful if there is a regulatory organization and/or requirements that must be met for each grade. Otherwise, anyone can label their product with whatever grade they want its kind of like essential oil companies that states their oils are certified 100% grade therapeutic oil. There isn't a governed entity that grades essential oils and all essential companies are none as certifiable because it's their products.

I'll try to do my best in relaying the findings

Human Hair extensions are measured in Grades and the lower the grade, the cheaper the price and the lowest longevity of the hair extensions.

Grade 'A' Is said to be mixed human hair where the cuticles have been stripped and replaced by a silicone coating for shine hair. It could be mixed with natural fallen hair and animal hair. This hair does not have a long life lasting on average 1 month with extra care and minimal use.

Grade 'AA' is when Human hair that has been subjected to more basic production processes than higher graded hair but remains a top seller in the hair industry due to its low prices. Grade AA hair will last 2-3 months on average when maintained correctly.

Grade 'AAA' 3A human hair that is processed to create a more conditioned, longer lasting hair which can take more washes and stay looking soft, shiny and healthy for longer. Grade 3A hair will last 3-4 months on average when maintained correctly.

Grade 'AAAA' or 4A human hair goes through higher and longer quality control process to ensure it stays soft, shiny & tangle free for longer and extended wear. It is very strong and durable and will last 4-6 months on average when maintained correctly.

Grade 'AAAAA' or 5A the highest quality processed 100% Remy human hair that is available. It has such strength that it is similar in condition to Virgin hair. The AAAAA grade hair started life as Virgin hair which has then been gently colored to bring a wide variety of natural looking European colors. The ratio of long hairs is extremely high and it is often double drawn so there will be no tapering towards the ends. It will remain soft, sleek and healthy for 9-12 months when maintained.

Virgin hair (**'AAAAA' Grade**) is the best quality hair your money can buy. The name 'Virgin' means that the hair is still in its pure form and it hasn't been dyed/bleached or chemically treated in any way. It is completely un-processed and has just been cleaned before being made into weft bundles. Because of this the hair stays softer which lasts much longer with great shine. Virgin hair is paramount of the human hair world. It is extremely strong, durable and can last 1-2 years if maintained correctly.

Now when you purchase weave you may see other grading system for example

Actually, **_Grade super A+_**, is the best quality, but it is much more expensive than other grades because it is used best raw hair with double drawn. Mostly grade AAA+, Grade AAA and Grade AA are very good quality raw hair with good prices.

'**_Grade B_**' the more basic 100% human hair that has been subjected to more basic production processes than higher graded hair but remains a top seller in the hair industry due to its low prices, it is said that 'Grade B' hair will last 1-2 months.

'**_Grade A series_**' is 100% Remy human hair that is processed to create a more conditioned stronger hair with more vibrant colors, it can take more washes and stay looking top quality for longer, it is said that 'Grade A' hair will last at least 6-8 months.

'**_Grade Super A_**' human hair is the most premium Remy of all hairs, its cuticles are left intact for maximum manageability, it has such strength that it is similar in condition to European hair and will last for 10-12 months.

From Goddessweave.com states, "from 5a to 10a it is impossible to grade virgin hair. It is not universal. At the time just a few years ago the highest quality of hair was 3A and then Chinese companies came along increasing the grading system from 4a to 10a. It has been copied and reworded ever since and now has become acceptable to the consumer as a grading system." So whichever grading system you use please make sure it appears natural.

C hapter 4 Problem Hair Issues

I just recently spoke to an old friend about her grand-daughter's hair issue and she told me that she wanted something that would grow making her grand-daughter's hair thicker. She also told me that she had eczema around her scalp and in her head. One of the things that I always try to mention that eczema is a signal that something is wrong internally. The issue has finally worked its way externally. This is not a Duh moment and its very critical information.

For example, when I moved to Lubbock, Texas in my mid-twenties I began to have serious allergy issues such as uncontrollable hay fever, hives, and sinus issues. I would break into hives from club or cigarette smoke. There were times it seem like taking in a breath of fresh air would make me miserable and I would be afraid to go almost anywhere. Several times I was sent to the emergency room because I would swell up like a handful of Mylar balloons at a six year's old birthday party. I believe this was the initial sign that something internally was going on. But, most of us only view allergies as topical and not internal. So, I always suggest paying attention to your diet to notice when the eczema is most active, such as change of seasons, food, and physical activities. Trust me it's not easy especially with all the junk combinations of toxic food that are available to us may take a life time trying to reconnect to nature the right way. Eventually, after several decades I finally got the hives under control but not before I ended up with eczema on my right foot, and bronchitis that happened on an average of six times a year.

When the diagnosis for Interstitial Cystitis entered into my life I had been suffering and going to the doctors for allergies, acid reflux, and IBS since 1994 and did not get the proper diagnosis until 2008. It took the toxic build up bananas along with other chemical based preservatives to have a radical reaction in my bladder for me to pay attention. The bottom line the allergies, acid reflux and IBS were signs of something much more serious. This indeed created supersized histamine mass growing in my bladder from the annoyance of nitrates and preservatives that had been accumulating in my system. Now with that being said back to your hair I do not believe that a product that helps to control any hair or body issue will work properly if there isn't a change in lifestyle or diet. I suggested to my friend before we try to make the hair grow lets heal it first. What do you mean heal it? If you cut your arm and depending on how deeply you will either have a scratch or a wound. You would not leave it unattended. Some type of antiseptic and maybe a bandage will dress the problem but, it will get some attention because you need it to be healed. It's the same thing with your hair. Your skin is the largest organ on your body and hair is the crowning glory of healthy skin. It is said in some scientific realms that hair on the knuckles of your fingers and toes mean that you have good circulation. I know at this point you're looking at your hand and foot but, don't worry. Let's continue on so, we now know we need to heal the scalp. The first step is not using heavy hair dressing creams because your hair needs to air and be free of unwanted un-needed solvents. I suggest first to use a shampoo that was made just for eczema and psoriasis issues that are free of paraben, dyes, sulfates, and alcohol.

This brings me to what type of hair issues that is out there:

Dandruff

Dandruff is a condition of the scalp that causes flakes of skin to appear. It occurs when the renewed skin is produced faster than the old dead skin can be expelled from the scalp which is marked by itching and flaking. This flaking is the result of more skin being shed. Dandruff can become a nuisance and embarrassing as it begins to shed on clothing or just by combing or brushing your hair. Proper care and treatment with non-drying shampoos can help tremendously.

I know in the past this was a big issue for me especially when I had relaxed hair that would always itch and when I combed or brushed there would be flakes of dried skin in the bathroom sink and on my shoulders. Of course, I tried everything from *Head & Shoulders* to *T-Gel* shampoo to no avail but, I will say once I did the transition learning what shampoo worked best for my natural mane. It wasn't a commercial shampoo but homemade. I am happy to say I might occasionally have dandruff but I do not have that overwhelming urge to scratch my head.

Alopecia

Alopecia is the medical term for hair loss. There are several patterns of natural and disease related hair loss. Hair loss may also be caused by several drugs and medications.

Types of Alopecia and symptoms

- The commonest type of hair loss is male-pattern baldness. This type of hair loss is typically caused by the effects of hormones. This is also termed androgenic or androgenetic alopecia as the cause lies in androgens of male sex hormones. There is a pattern of receding hairline along with thinning of hair over the crown.
- Female pattern baldness – there is thinning of hair over the top of the head.
- Alopecia areata – this is also termed patchy baldness as there are patches of baldness that come and go. This may commonly affect teenagers and young adults but may affect a person of any age. Alopecia areata is commonly caused due to a problem in the immune system. The condition may sometimes run in families.
- Scarring alopecia – this is mainly caused after a scar over the skin. This type of alopecia is called cicatricial alopecia. The hair follicles that hold the roots of the hair may be completely destroyed. This means that the hair would not grow back at the areas affected. Some diseases and disorders also cause scarring alopecia. These include lichen planus, injury, discoid lupus etc.
- Anagen effluvium is a more widespread hair loss that may affect the whole body apart from the scalp. This is caused most commonly due to cancer chemotherapy.
- Telogen effluvium - leads to thinning of hair all over the body rather than baldness in patches. This may be the result of stress of some medications

I see quite a few clients that suffer from alopecia due to hormonal or medical issues and it is alarming because quite a few are African

American women who continually stress out their hair with inferior products and harsh chemicals. Sometimes, it seems like a no win situation because you are losing your hair and you need to cover the loss by wearing either wigs or weaves but these factor in as well to loss of hair. Wigs promote hair loss around the edges and keeping your hair from breathing while weaves are just a mess by taking out more hair with glue and braids. So your once gorgeous hair is getting a double whammy.

Balding

I definitely do not want to overlook the men. It would seem in this day and age that shaving the head bald is popular and very attractive but, there are a few men that still want to have a nice clean cut or fade. They also can suffer premature male baldness. Even though as a woman we might not understand the big deal for a man since hair is touted as a woman's crown of glory that men too can be ashamed. It's not something to be ashamed of but something that gives you a moment to take a break and step back to see what changes in your life can result in better hair.

I had a male client that was in his thirties that had a bald spot behind his ear with the possible appearance of ringworm and then he had thinning hair on top. After talking to him about baldness in his family, his age, testosterone, and his diet I felt that he was a prime candidate for a specific balding men formula. Usually, I inform clients that you can expect results anywhere from two months to a six month period. The gentlemen sent me a before and after pictures after the first week. Then a month later he sent another picture which I was astounded. But, you have to understand he was serious in what he was doing. Exercising and eating right plays a very important role in your hair health.

I just don't want you to assume that balding is just for men. Over the last decade I have met many women that are absolutely bald under the wigs unfortunately these women are in their late sixties to early seventies. Don't get me wrong I have friends that are younger or close to my age that are experiencing some serious hair trauma. I suspect that many of these types of hair issues are results of hormonal problems such as I mentioned earlier hysterectomies. Hysterectomies play havoc on a woman's health from circulatory, thyroids, immune, and hormonal system. Our bodies have to reorganize or reconstruct another alternative way of sustaining our health which can result in a poor quality of life in the long run. Other reasons can include the use of continued relaxers in your youth to adulthood which have weakened hair follicles over time. But whatever the reasons which can be hard to determine awareness has to be brought to the forefront. Usually when a woman experience hair loss especially around the edges or the nape of the neck we can look at that as thinning or alopecia. The culprit could be anywhere from stress to hair glues. Usually if a woman begins to experience hair loss in the middle of her head it may be a sign of premature baldness which sometimes known as a hereditary issue. We know that hair loss can be problematic but reducing the age factor in the body by keeping healthy cell functions in check can delay hereditary factors. Understanding proper eating, hair stressors, exercising and supplementation can helps us knowing our bodies better.

Even though there are allopathic drugs to help fight hair loss or balding they are not always effective. There are many pharmaceutical drugs that have the potential to stimulate hair loss which are also known to control hypertension as well but what are you doing to your body if you don't suffer from hypertension and you are prescribing to one of these medicines for hair loss?

That's when naturopathic assistance comes knocking per se at your door. Essential oils can help with alopecia, thinning hair, or even baldness without having to worry about unwanted side effects. Just remember all plant life have chemical reactions and you may have a potential to have an allergic reaction as such but, it's safer than having an allergic reaction to synthetic chemicals that you cannot even pronounce. Most medicines are made to treat a specific but herbs or essential oils are made to treat the whole body by bringing it back into balance.

Falling Hair

When I first began my transition from relaxed back to natural I noticed I was losing quite a bit of hair. I can't even describe it as shedding because it was so much. It gave me tremendous concerns because I always had thick hair. I knew that I was battling forces that I didn't understand trying to keep a head full of hair. I was on one particular medication that specifically stated that if you were African American you would incur hair loss. According to Health.Com states, "thinning hair and hair loss are also common in women, and no less demoralizing. Reasons can range from the simple and temporary a vitamin deficiency—to the more complex, like an underlying health condition. It can be from physical stress to pregnancy. Of course the problem is to find the underlying cause and fix it.

For example, I had a client that was suffering from hair loss when she came to visit. She did not wear a wig when she came but had on a cap. I asked her to let me see her hair, and it was thick but you could tell that it had some damage especially split ends and upper breakage. Fortunately, we weren't too deep in her history before the culprit to her hair loss reared its ugly head. She had lost her father a few years ago and was still coping. The stress of the loss of a loved one took its toll on her head. Sometimes, we already know the answers but need confirmation with a complete total stranger. We talked or rather I ran my mouth but, it was healing for both of us. A few months passed from that wonderful spiritual healing that when I saw her she was radiant and hair was beautiful.

I know there are many other hair issues that can be addressed but I only addressed the top complaints that I deal with from day to day with my own clients. My suggestion for you is to seek out a professional dermatologist, physician or naturopath to help you resolve your hair problems. It could be deeper than just your follicles.

Chapter 5 Knowing Your Products

Here we will go over briefly the definitions of our hair products even though we may have a clear understanding of their position in regards to hair care we can look at these products closely later on in the book . I have to say first that organic products are the best way to go to ensure healthy hair free of aluminum, dyes, alcohol, parabens, and sodium laureate that may have carcinogenic properties.

Shampoo definition by Wikipedia states, shampoo is a product that is used for the removal of oils, dirt, skin particles, dandruff, environmental pollutants and other contaminant particles that gradually build up in hair. The goal of using shampoo is to remove the unwanted build-up without stripping out so much sebum as to make hair unmanageable. Using shampoo also allows the hair to be nourished and healthy.

Shampooing is essential for cleansing the scalp but with today's commercial shampoos of sodium laureates and other drying agents you have to be careful of toxic buildup that leave your hair dry, damaged, and unhealthy. Look for shampoos that do not carry SLS (sodium lauryl sulfates) which can causes rashes on back of neck, shoulders and also as an eye irritant. Alternatives are castile soap, soap wort or herbal infusions. May not foam as what you're accustomed to but is highly effective and beneficial.

Conditioners definition by Wise Geek states, Hair conditioner is a hair care product that is applied after shampooing in order to condition the hair. It is most useful for people with dry or damaged hair, as people with naturally oily hair may find conditioner weighs their hair down rather than improves the overall look and feel of it. There are wide ranges of hair conditioning products, including those you rinse out, leave in, or spray on. I suggest to hair clients especially Alopecia sufferers to condition hair first to help stimulate circulation, prepare the hair, and to remove heavy residue on scalp before shampoo. The next step is to follow up with a gentle shampoo and a nice vinegar rinse. Rinses will leave the hair with shine and luster.

Moisturizers definition is that it must improve or maintain hydration levels of hair. Proper levels of moisture help maintain the keratin structure and mechanical integrity of the hair. Folks that have kinky hair normally lack moisture thus needing moisturizing almost daily. There are a wide variety of moisturizers on the market just make sure that none contain drying chemicals such as alcohol; or BHA (butylated hydroxyanisole) and BHT (butylated hydroxytoluene) which can cause allergies of the skin and possible carcinogenic to humans . Once again your best alternatives are moisturizers that have been certified organic and you are familiar with the ingredients.

Rinses – When I mention rinses I am not referring to what you do after you shampoo and condition your hair. Most of us associate rinsing with water and we're done. Rinses maybe a new thing for most Americans but it is very popular in other countries. A great hair rinse gives nutrients to the hair, shine and moisture and perhaps can prevent graying as well. What? It prevents graying so let's learn a little a bit about rinses.

Rinses are the finale after shampooing and conditioning your hair, rinses can add luster and clean up and out a lot of product residual by making your hair squeaky clean and healthy as well. Especially vinegar rinses are known to do very well on all hair types for its ability to draw out cleanse and heal hair shafts. Don't get Rinses confused with semi-rinses which are mostly adding color to your hair that washes out over time.

Teas – Hair Teas are very new to the hair scene as well but they have been around since ancient times for medicinal purposes such as lice, fungus, for hygiene purposes of cleansing the hair, and for cosmetic purposes for scenting and coloring the hair. Hair teas are great for giving your hair the extra nutrients and benefits as well. Even if you have colored hair the teas help to prolong the color too. Hair teas are fun because you can boil the teas and pour the cool tea over your head as your final rinse giving your hair shine, luster, strength and a natural fragrance as well without any harsh chemicals.

Detangler- I believe every head that has hair should have a detangler in the cabinet or bathroom. Many people with long hair or those who have dry curly hair suffer from strands of hair that knot up and become a ball of agony. When this happens the hair can become damaged more in the process of trying to remove the knotted strands. Detanglers help to soften the knots per se to make it easier to brush or comb out the offending knot. A detangler is like a conditioner that has a polymer or oil base that can acidify the hair. Its primary function is to smooth the hair so it can become free of its static cling and hair balls. Some conditioners work well as a detangler also. Look for ingredients such as carrier oils, aloes, glycerin and water in the product as a useful detangler.

Sealants – sealants go hand in hand with moisturizing. Especially, if you have dry hair a great sealant is very necessary. The main goal of sealing the hair is to trap the moisture in your cuticles so it can't get out and excess moisture in the air can't get in.

I've listed several great sealants

Shea Butter Oil has natural antioxidant and anti inflammatory properties that acts as a great protection for sun damaged hair

Olive Oil is great for dry scalp sufferers and helps with maintain healthy hair.

Coconut Oil has so many great benefits that using it on your hair is a must. It helps with shine and thinning hair.

Grapeseed Oil reduces hair loss, strengthens, reduces dermatitis and dandruff.

Aloe Vera Gel is a must go to providing you with plenty of benefits to cleanse, protect, and nourish hair.

Castor Oil nourishes the scalp and strengthens the roots.

Emollients- Emollients are just another fancy name for moisturizers. Emollients come in many forms from lotions, creams, oils, and ointments. The purpose of emollients is to keep your skin in our case your hair from drying out, preventing breakage, reducing itching, and giving moisture to hair.

Humectants -Humectants are used in hair and skin care products to promote moisture retention. They have the ability to attract water from the atmosphere. This ability between the humectants and water improves moisture retention by minimizing water loss due to evaporation. Because of their water-binding abilities humectants are ideal for dry, thirsty hair. Some natural humectants are vegetable glycerin, honey, and agave nectar.

Chapter 6 Knowing Essential Oils

In many of our organic hair care products there will be essential oils or extracts. Essential oils are like concentrated oils of particular herbs or plants that have been specially formulated and blended to give you the optima care in hair care products. Essential oils are natural oils that are typically obtained by distillation and having the characteristic fragrance of the plant or other source from which it is extracted. There are many essential oils that work well on all hair types and are incorporated in many commercialized products as botanicals. My opinion to go organic as much as possible but if you opt for regular hair care products make sure you are getting your monies worth. There is a particular company's shampoo and conditioner that markets Kukui oil as its top billing but after looking at the ingredients it is the last on the list. Which in the past means the last ingredient is the least amount present. I believe that representation is still accepted today!

The categories below are broken down to hair condition. Pay attention because some herbs may repeat in each category and others may not. If an herb is not mentioned in your category than do not use it.

For Normal Hair

The best essential oils are:

Lavender (Lavendula Augustofolia) is great at reducing excess sebum on skin and hair loss

Lemon (Citrus lemon) it's known to clean toxins from all parts of the body especially hair and skin

Eucalyptus Lemon (Corymbia citriodora) promotes growth and stimulates hair

Parsley (Petroselinum crispum) prevents hair loss

Geranium (Pelargonium graveolens) helps to calm and distress hair follicles and scalp

Carrot (Daucus Carota) helps soften, promotes growth and great for dermatitis

Rosemary (Rosmarinus officinalis) stimulates hair growth

Cedarwood (Cedras atlantica) promotes circulation

Thyme (Thymus vulgaris) antimicrobial and antiseptic

Clary Sage (Petroselinum crispum) prevents hair loss

Dry Hair

Lavender (Lavendula Augustofolia) is great at reducing excess sebum on skin and hair loss

Rosemary (Rosmarinus officinalis) stimulates hair growth

Geranium (Pelargonium graveolens) helps to calm and distress hair follicles and scalp

Birch (Betula lenta) is excellent to help promote hair growth

Carrot (Daucus Carota) helps soften, promotes growth and great for dermatitis

Parsley (Petroselinum crispum) prevents hair loss

Yarrow (Achillea millefolium) promotes hair growth

Sandalwood (Santalum albumis) promotes healthy hair, adds moisture

Oily /Greasy Hair

Rosemary (Rosmarinus officinalis) stimulates hair growth

Lavender (Lavendula Augustofolia) is great at reducing excess sebum on skin and hair loss

Cypress (Cypressus sempervirens) alleviates dandruff, hair loss and promotes growth

Lemon (Citrus lemon) it's known to clean toxins from all parts of the body especially hair and skin

Eucalyptus Lemon (Corymbia citriodora) promotes growth and stimulates hair

Pimento Berry (Pimenta officinalis) stimulates hair growth and circulation

Birch (Betula lenta) is excellent to help promote hair growth

Basil (Ocimum basilcum) relieves dandruff

Sage (Salvia officinalis) dandruff and hair loss

Thyme (Thymus vulgaris) antimicrobial and antiseptic

Yarrow (Achillea millefolium) promotes hair growth

Peppermint (Mentha piperita) eczema, psoriasis, dandruff and hair loss

Fragile Hair

Parsley (Petroselinum crispum) prevents hair loss

Lavender (Lavendula Augustofolia) is great at reducing excess sebum on skin and hair loss

Chamomile (Matricaria chamomilla) great for preventing or reducing hair loss

Birch (Betula lenta) is excellent to help promote hair growth

Thyme (Thymus vulgaris) antimicrobial and antiseptic helping to keep scalp clean

Calendula (Calendula arvensis) helps to bring out luster and shine

Carrot (Daucus Carota) helps soften, promotes growth and great for dermatitis

Sandalwood (Santalum albumis) promotes healthy hair, adds moisture

Clary Sage (Petroselinum crispum) prevents hair loss

If you notice that Rosemary and Lavender are primarily in all hair type groups it's because you cannot go wrong with these two because of their beneficial hair properties. Lavender helps to calm the hair follicles reducing redness and inflammation as well. Rosemary is soothing helping to alleviate flaky itchy scalps. As you may notice some herbs listed in the Essential Oil section are highly concentrated. If you would like to make a shampoo or a rinse using some of the essential oils make sure that they are diluted in carrier oil for protection.

I hope this helps for when you are looking for that natural organic product and you know the truth is out there for you to discover more about hazardous chemicals in your hair care products. Remember a Wiser You is a Healthier You!

Chapter 7 Knowing Herbs & Supplements

I use a lot of fresh and dried herbs for hair care products whether it's infusing with carrier oils, boiling fresh or dried herbs with distilled water to create an infusion, Herbs for your hair are great and easy if you don't have money available for expensive hair care products. The fun part you probably can easily find in your kitchen spice rack herbs to use to improve the quality of your hair, shine and texture.

Here are the Top Ten Herbs for your hair

Aloe Vera (*Aloe barbadensis)* When directly applied on the hair, aloe Vera promotes hair growth by stimulating blood circulation along the scalp. Massage aloe Vera on your scalp and this also restores the hair's PH balance and opens up your scalp's blocked pores that will allow growth of hair follicles. All Mrs Jacks shampoos contain 100 % Organic Aloe Vera

Burdock (*Arctium lappa*) this herb definitely has its benefits to people suffering from hair loss. Burdock actually promotes healthy hair by improving the circulation of blood to the hair follicle and in relieving scalp irritations. Burdock contains high levels of essential fatty acids and phytosterol compounds that are known to be effective reversing and reducing hair thinning. Phytosterol is actually one of the most potent ingredients of many hair restoration products in the market today.

Horsetail (*Equisetum)* is called such because of its long brush-like features; horsetail's potent ingredient is silica which is responsible for strengthening bones, nails and hair. It restores brittle hair to keep it from breaking or thinning thereby preventing further hair loss. Because of its hair loss remedy properties, horsetail is often found in many conditioning products to fortify and repair hair

Ginkgo Biloba (*Ginkgo Biloba*) which is its scientific name but also known as Maiden Hair is like aloe Vera, ginkgo biloba is said to increase blood flow to the brain to correct any nutritional deficiencies to hair follicles. As a result, this has likewise become a popular herbal remedy for hair re-growth.

Lavender (*Lavendula Augustofolia*) lavender has been widely used by herbal practitioners in encouraging hair growth and in preventing baldness. Lavender is anti-bacterial as well as anti-fungal so it helps to heal and soothe skin infections as well as in relieving dandruff. When used regularly, lavender is capable of preventing hair loss as well as in ensuring significant re-growth of hair. There are many products that carries lavender such as body washes to soaps as well as hair care products because of its calming and relaxing effects for preventing the occurrence of stress, insomnia and depression which are widely considered as common causes of alopecia or hair loss.

Chinese Ginseng *(Panax Ginseng)* Hair growth is just one of the medicinal values of this popular ancient Chinese herb. Applied as a tonic or shampoo, ginseng is often used to address male baldness by nourishing and strengthening the hair.

Peppermint (*Mentha piperita*)
I know many folks love peppermint because it is one of the few herbs besides lavender that people are willing to expose themselves to. It is regarded as a wisely used commercialized product whether as oil, tea, medicinal, or other cosmetic purposes. Peppermint oil also makes an excellent hair grower because it promotes hair growth by stimulating the growth of hair follicles. When applied as oil, peppermint offers cooling and soothing effects to the scalp and it is also capable of binding the hair roots as well as in encouraging better circulation to the scalp. According to studies, enhanced circulation significantly affects the process of hair growing.

Rosemary (*Rosmarinus Officinalis*) for centuries, rosemary has been widely used as a solution to hair loss, hair thinning balding or receding hairline. It actually works by stimulating the circulation in the scalp thereby resulting to hair growth. This works best when added to olive oil and applied as oil. Regular application of rosemary oil even helps in preventing premature graying as well as in treating dry and flaky scalp. It also helps with itching, flakiness and dry scalp. It is an excellent conditioner. Furthermore, rosemary works by strengthening and nourishing the hair follicles starting from the shaft.

Saw Palmetto (*Serenoa repens)* is another ancient remedy which is thought to cure balding by preventing the conversion of testosterone into DHT. DHT is responsible for receding hairline in both men and women. It is often recommended to be used together with Stinging Nettle (see below) which serves the same function.

Stinging Nettle (*Urtica Diocia)* abundantly found in North America, stinging nettle is a potent plant known for its hair growing benefits. Its reported mechanism of action is by preventing the conversion of testosterone hormones into dihydrotestosterone (DHT). According to studies, excessive production of DHT normally triggers hair loss. Although stinging nettle can be purchased in capsule or pill form, stinging nettle can also be applied as oil and I use stinging nettle leaf in some of my shampoos and it is really effective for parasites as well as alopecia.

Having a head of healthy hair is just as having a healthy body and healthy skin. They are all a product of what you consume externally and internally. Poor diets, poor health, heavy medications, abusive chemicals will cause your hair to change or even fall out. Getting plenty of sleep and eating plenty of fresh fruits and vegetables can help tremendously along with cutting down on stimulants such as coffee, tea, sodas and alcohol.

Eating the proper diet can be difficult especially in this day and age with fast and processed foods around every corner sometimes can be fighting a battle uphill.

Get involved with vitamins that can help restore and grow your hair

Starting off with Vitamin B and your best bet is B12. B's unlike the other vitamins have so many from B1 to even a B17 can you're your body immensely. B's are the building blocks of your body.

Another wonderful vitamin is E because E is great for your skin and excellent for all hair types as well. You can take it as a supplement or buy vitamin E oil and add it to your hair care products. I personally suggest that if you are battling hair issues not to bother with a

multivitamin containing these vitamins because you're getting the recommended daily allowances which is based upon a healthy lifestyle. The next important vitamin is not actually a vitamin but a hormone that is encouraged by the sun which is vitamin D. This fantastic vitamin that we mostly look at with calcium gets ignored in the hair care industry but it is known to promote healthy hair follicles.

Another great hair suggestion that I definitely want to include is Biotin. For it is the most known supplement for growing nails, hair and having beautiful skin. So make sure if you're not eating right and you cannot get these vitamins in your body daily then try to incorporate vitamins to your regiment paying attention when you notice changes in your hair. There are more vitamins out there to help you obtain a beautiful mane so, do a little research. You can benefit from those supplements for not only your beauty care needs but for your health also. Remember a healthy you is a wiser you!

Chapter 8 Knowing Carrier Oils

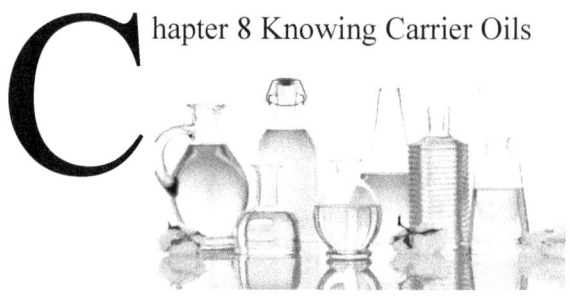

There are many types of carrier oils on the market and with the growing hair industry commercializing on new specialty oils of the month that tout that they are better. Carrier oils are great for helping to carry the essential oil process because some essential oils are strong and dilution is required. Also, carrier oils are great for softening hard butters as well as great for cooking. There are many other benefits of carrier oils and we are going to go over a few for the best carrier oils for your hair type.

The best carrier oil for **Normal hair** is

Sweet Almond Oil (*Prunus dulcis*) is obtained from the kernel and very pale yellow. It is rich in protein, vitamins and minerals. Can be used 100 percent as base oil for all skin types. The primary benefit of sweet almond oil is as a sealant and hair protector because it is light, non-greasy, fast absorbing oil that conditions the hair.

Peach Kernel Oil (*Prunus persica*) is rich in vitamins, polyunsaturated fatty acids, proteins and minerals. Yellow in color and is great for all skin types. It acts as an emollient. By coating the hair shaft, it retains natural color and chemically applied color, making color treatments last longer.

Borage Seed Oil (*Borago officinalis*) is obtained from the seeds and is pale yellow in color and contains gamma linolenic acid, vitamin and minerals. Borage seed oil is great for all skin types and great for inflamed follicles.

Evening Primrose Oil *(Oenothera biennes L)* is found from the flower of the same name; it is pale yellow in color and contains gamma linolenic acid, vitamins and minerals. It's excellent in the treatment of eczema and psoriasis. It can be used on the scalp and around hairline to alleviate dermatitis issues.

Hemp oil *(Cannabis sativa)* can be used to beautify your hair from within, as well as from without. The oil is rich in essential fatty acids, along with vitamins and protein. Hemp oil is good for people with all hair and skin types. The oil is also a natural moisturizer that boosts scalp health, shoring up the intercellular matrix, which protects against moisture loss. Hemp oil has vitamin E, along with high essential fatty acid content.

Tamanu Oil *(Calophyllum inophyllum)* is obtained from the kernel, green in color, and contains lipids and great for all hair types. Lipids are any of class of organic compounds that are fatty acids or their derivatives and are insoluble in water but soluble in organic solvents. They include many natural oils, waxes, and steroids.

Extra Virgin Olive Oil *(Olea europaea)*- even though pure olive oil is okay but the first fruits of the pressed olives is the best. So stick with extra virgin olive oil in your hair care regiment. This oil is a stable for a lot of curly girl regimens. Olive oil provides long last moisturizing benefits and can help with healthy hair and skin. Add olive oil to for deep conditioning treatments.

Dry Hair

This is a special category because of my own personal hair issue. After so many meds for several years my hair took a turn for the worse in which moisturizing became the main concern for keeping my hair healthy. It is a difficult process so, for dry hair folks I gave this section some extra attention because there are plenty of wonderful oils that can help.

Apricot Kernel Oil (*Prunus armeniaca*) comes from the kernels of apricot. Apricot oil is a great source for vitamin A, E and minerals. This oil can be used to help seal ends and to help prevent split ends. It's also great to treat dandruff and helps with inflammation of the scalp. It gives shine and moisture to lack luster dry hair.

Sesame Seed Oil (*Sesamum indicum*) is chocked for of goodness that contains minerals, vitamins, proteins, amino acids and lecithin. It is dark yellow in color and great for all skin types. It is great for treating eczema and psoriasis. It is light antibacterial oil that is great for dry scalps. It penetrates quickly and nourishes the hair. Be advised that regular use will cause the hair to darken.

Jojoba Oil (*Simmondsia chinensis*) is obtained from the beans and contains protein, minerals, and a waxy substance that mimics collagen. It is yellow in color and great for all skin types. It is a great moisturizer for hair.

Borage Seed Oil (*Borago officinalis*) is obtained from the seeds and is pale yellow in color and contains gamma linolenic acid, vitamin and minerals. Great for all skin types and great for inflamed follicles.

 Evening Primrose *(Oenothera biennes L)* is found from the flower of the same name; it is pale yellow in color and contains gamma linolenic acid, vitamins and minerals. It's excellent in the treatment of eczema and psoriasis and is used at 10 percent dilution. . It can be used on the scalp to control eczema and psoriasis around the hairline. It is also good for alleviating any other dermatitis issues.

Peach Kernel Oil (*Prunus persica*) is rich in vitamins, polyunsaturated fatty acids, proteins and minerals. Yellow in color and is great for all skin types. By gently coating the hair shaft, peach kernel oil protects hair from environmental conditions such as sun, wind, rain and pollution. Coating the hair shaft with light oil also deters frizz and helps define curl patterns

Argan Oil (*Argania spinosa*) is expressed from the seeds and contains unsaturated fatty acids, Vitamin E, squalene and sterols. Repairs damaged hair. Moisturizes instantly, and prevents split ends while restoring shine. Increases hair growth and helps control, cure, and prevent dry and itchy scalp. Argan oil is lightweight and is a great finishing product for shiny hair and to tame frizz. Apply from the ends of your hair up to your scalp.

Tamanu Oil (*Calophyllum inophyllum*) is obtained from the kernel, green in color, and contains lipids and great for all hair types. It's also known as a great healer for skin issues.

Sunflower Oil (*Helianthus annuus*) contains vitamins and minerals, great for all skin types, pale yellow in color, used at 100 percent and is excellent for fine or oily hair.

Avocado (*Persea Americana*) is obtained from the fruit and is dark green in color. It contains vitamins A, D, and E, potassium, protein, fatty acids, and lecithin as well. It is excellent for all skin types and great for eczema and dehydrated skin. It can be used as a great moisturizer with anti-aging benefits. It is very nourishing to the hair.

Neem seed oil (*Azadirachta indica*) is anti-fungal and anti-bacterial. In addition, neem seed oil can treat dry and itchy scalp. Its properties will help to cleanse the scalp of dandruff, flakes, itchiness, and buildup.

Hemp Oil (*Cannabis sativa*) adds gloss and manageability to hair. Loaded with essential fatty acids that moisturizes and replenishes the skin as well as the hair. It is great for dry scalp and damaged hair

Kukui Oil (*Aleurites moluccans)* the Kukui nut tree is the official tree of Hawaii, and has been used by natives for hundreds of years. Kukui nut oil contains high levels of the essential fatty acids linoleic, alpha-linolenic, antioxidants, as well as Vitamins A, C and E. This oil is readily absorbed into the skin, can also use it for an oil treatment on dry hair and scalp. Kukui oil is expeller expressed from the nuts, and is light yellow with an amber tint. It has a limited shelf life so store in a cool, dry place away from heat and light.

Oily/Greasy

Evening Primrose Oil *(Oenothera biennes L*) is found from the flower of the same name; it is pale yellow in color and contains gamma linolenic acid, vitamins and minerals. It's excellent in the treatment of eczema and psoriasis.

Borage Seed Oil (*Borago officinalis*) is obtained from the seeds and is pale yellow in color and contains gamma linolenic acid, vitamin and minerals. Great for all hair and skin types because its benefits for dermatitis problems, and it is anti-inflammatory, antioxidant, and acts as an emollient .

Sesame Seed Oil (*Sesamum indicum*) is chocked for of goodness such it contains minerals, vitamins, proteins, amino acids and lecithin. It is dark yellow in color and great for all skin types.

 Peach Kernel Oil (*Prunus persica*) is rich in vitamins, polyunsaturated fatty acids, proteins and minerals. Yellow in color, great for all skin types and helps to nourish oily hair.

Aragan Oil (*Argania spinosa*) is expressed from the seeds and contains unsaturated fatty acids, Vitamin E, squalene, and sterols. Repairs damaged hair. Moisturizes instantly, and prevents split ends while restoring shine. Increases hair growth and helps control, cure, and prevent dry and itchy scalp.

Tamanu Oil (*Calophyllum inophyllum*) is obtained from the kernel, green in color, and contains lipids and great for all hair types.

Jojoba Oil (*Simmondsia chinensis*) is similar to the hair's natural oil and inhibits overproduction of the sebaceous glands making it great for oily scalps.

Fragile Hair

I would like to give special attention to this category by including baldness, alopecia, and thinning hair. You must factor in diet, heredity, and medical problems for the causes of these particular hair issues. Seek the advice of a medical professional when confronting with hair loss issues.

Jojoba Oil (*Simmondsia chinensis*) is obtained from the beans and contains protein, minerals, and a waxy substance that mimics collagen. It is yellow in color and great for all skin types. Jojoba Oil moisturizes the hair and is great for hair loss caused by breakage.

Borage Seed Oil (*Borago officinalis*) is obtained from the seeds and is pale yellow in color and contains gamma linolenic acid, vitamin and minerals. Great for all skin types and it has been known to slow down hair loss

Sweet Almond Oil (*Prunus dulcis*) is obtained from the kernel and very pale yellow. It is rich in protein, vitamins and minerals. Can be used 100 percent as base oil for all skin and hair types.

Evening Primrose *(Oenothera biennes L)* is found from the flower of the same name; it is pale yellow in color and contains gamma linolenic acid, vitamins and minerals. It's excellent in the treatment of eczema and psoriasis which can help reduce stress on hair and strengthen follicles.

Peach Kernel Oil (*Prunus persica*) is rich in vitamins, polyunsaturated fatty acids, proteins and minerals. Yellow in color and is great for all skin types. It is light oil that is easy to wash out and it doesn't weigh down thin hair.

Tamanu Oil (*Calophyllum inophyllum*) is obtained from the kernel, green in color, and contains lipids and great for all hair types.

Alma Oil (*Phyllanthus emblica*) is Ayurvedic herbal oil made from Indian gooseberry and is used to promote hair health and hair loss. Daily scalp massages with Alma oil will not only help with dry scalp, but aid in hair growth.

Castor Oil (*Ricinus communis*) made from the castor beans can be used to help thicken hair and works as wonderful humectants. It attracts and retains moisture to the hair, making it a great emollient when used with other oils.

Coconut Oil (*Cocos nucifera*) is a light moisturizer that can be used to moisturize your hair, body, and skin. Coconut oil is also a great oil to use as pre-shampoo conditioning and preparing the hair for the shampoo. The oil can be applied to your roots and detangle hair from ends to root. It can soften the hair, strengthen, and nourish damaged hair by preventing protein loss.

Emu Oil (*Dromaius Novae-Hollandiae*) is the oil of sterilized fat from Australian Emu birds. It is a highly penetrating and will not clog pores. It contains Vitamins A and E and has been used to reverse the effects of hair loss.

Wheat Germ Oil *(Triticum vulgare)* made from the germ or seed of the wheat has antioxidant and regenerative properties. It is loaded with vitamins and fatty acids such as Vitamins A, D, and E, protein, and essential fatty acids including Omega 6 and Omega 3, phosphatides, phytosterols, and octacosanol. It softens hair, soothes and nourishes irritated scalp, decreases thinning, and leaves a healthy scalp.

Even though there are numerous carrier oils popping up on the hair commercial scene the ones provided are the best known and experienced by the author. Know your health, hair and how it works and provide the correct hair care products for your hair so that you can receive the ultimate benefits of great hair.

C hapter 9 Knowing Butters

There are quite a few Butters that are made from fruit, beans, and seeds, and leaves of plants. Butters are produced by hydrogenating the cold pressed oil extracted from them. The most common butters are cocoa, mango, and Shea butter. Which are great for hair and skin care purposes but, fortunately, we are not limited to just these three butters. There's a whole new market on exotic butters ranging from inexpensive to expensive.

Mango Butter (*Mangifera Indica*)

Mangoes are a fruit that are native to Asia. Raw mango butter is rich in oleic acid, a mono-unsaturated omega-9 acid, and stearic acid, a saturated fatty acid. It comes from the kernel of the plant and it is rich in antioxidants such as A, C, and E. Mango butter is the fatty acid cold-pressed from mango seeds and . Its properties and even chemical structure are similar to cocoa and Shea butter, but Mango Butter is softer in texture than Shea and cocoa butter. The natural form of mango butter is semi-solid and non-greasy, and it is used as a moisturizer for hair to and soothes dry skin. It has a shelf life of two years.

Shea Butter (*Vitellaria paradoxa)*

The history of Shea as a commodity can be traced back to Ancient Egypt, where Shea butter continues to be used to protect the hair and skin. It is an off- white or ivory-colored fat extracted from the nut of the African Shea tree. Shea butter is a triglyceride (fat) derived mainly from stearic acid and oleic acid and because of that it is used today in some African countries as cooking oil. Nevertheless, in the hair care industry is acts as a sealant; it is great for holding conditioners and moisturizers in the hair. It should never be used on the hair dry. It is a heavy butter and is better used if warmed and parted on hair.

Cocoa Butter (*Theobroma cocao*)

Cocoa butter is a pale-yellow, edible vegetable fat extracted from the cocoa bean heavy and strong in scent but, is great for hair especially increasing manageability and moisture. It has excellent hydrating properties. Cocoa butter can help prevent hair loss due to breakage, alleviate scalp itching, irritation, and prevent chemical damage. It may increase volume and strength for those with fine hair as well. The amazing cocoa butter has been used as the main ingredient for making chocolate and because of its rich fragrance the more chemical richness of its benefits. It has a shelf life from 2 to 5 years.
It is best used as a pre conditioner on the hair and thin shampooed out after twenty minutes for maximum results.

Cupuacu Butter (*Theobroma Grandiflorum Seed Butter*)

Cupuacu Butter is obtained from the seeds of the Cupuacu tree that grows in the Brazilian Amazon. It is a rich exotic butter that is moist and creamy. It possesses a high capacity for water absorption which gives it superior moisturizing properties and is great for a natural UV-A and UV-B protectant therefore it is great as a sealant. The Cupuacu fruit has a nutritional content and is rich in antioxidants, vitamins B1, B2, B3, amino acids. It can be used to treat skin conditions such as eczema and dermatitis and adds shine and replenishes moisture in hair.

Coffee Bean Butter (*Capulus faba*)

Coffee Bean Butter is created by hydrogenating the oil that is pressed from roasted coffee beans along with soybean and/or sunflower oils. It has a fragrance of coffee and is rich, smooth and buttery. It is reminiscent of Cocoa butter and it is also excellent for skin irritation and skin inflammations. It has a natural protection from ultraviolet light and is becoming a popular ingredient in sunscreen products. Therefore it is great for dry skin. It has many antioxidants that are powerful against anti-irritation and anti-inflammatory properties which also makes it an excellent candidate to promote moisture in hair products.

Macadamia Nut Butter (*Macadamia integrifolia*)

Macadamia is a genus of four species of trees indigenous to Australia and if you are familiar with macadamia nuts and like them then you know they are a bit pricy but well deserving. The same goes for the butter which is a light butter and is great for treating dry hair and damaged skin. Since it is a wonderful moisturizer and rich in fatty acids especially palmitoleic acid. This particular acid is known for its anti-aging component therefore as mentioned making it excellent for the treating of dry hair and damaged skin.

MuruMuru Butter (*Astrocaryum MuruMuru*)

MuruMuru Butter is pressed from the reddish-orange fruits of the Astrocaryum MuruMuru tree. It is native to Brazil and other regions of the Amazon. Its unique composition of essential fatty acids and Pro-Vitamin A help restore elasticity to damaged and aging skin making it a highly suitable ingredient for use in anti-aging formulations. It is also soothing addition for products intended to heal dry and cracked skin, eczema and psoriasis. Its emollient properties, its natural gloss brings a desirable shine to dry, damaged hair and thus an excellent choice for shampoos, conditioners, and highly moisturizing hair. MuruMuru is part of The Fair Trade Commission because it is a handpicked fruit that helps sustain families inside the Forest.

Kokum Butter (*Garcinia indica*)

The kokum tree produces kiwi-sized fruit that is loaded with fatty acids and antioxidants. It is very similar to cocoa butter and can be chosen as a substitute for cocoa butter because of its uniform triglyceride composition. It is best used in combination with other butters and oils and is great for twists and twist outs. it has the ability to soften skin and heal ulcerations of lips, hands and soles of feet. Kokum Butter helps reduce degeneration of the skin cells and restores elasticity.

Tucuma Butter (*Astrocaryum Tucuma*)

Tucuma Butter is off white to light yellow in color and is considered a light butter rich in Vitamin A. It has high levels of lauric, Myristic, Oleic, and Fatty acid which makes it ideal to combat free radicals for lubricity, for both skin and hair, where it brings natural shine to dry, damaged, hair and a luminosity, and softness to skin. It serves as a great emollient. It has a light notable coffee fragrance and is pressed from the fruit (seeds) of the palm tree.

As butters are becoming more popular an increase in exotic butters are coming in the market. Familiarize yourself with their properties and benefits and make wise choices for your safety, health and lifestyle.

C hapter 10 Interpreting Labels

With consumer awareness labeling changes in the market can be overwhelming if you do not know the ploys and deceptions of business. I have read a lot of labels trying to make heads or tails of a myriad of ingredients and they all are confusing until I began making my own hair care products. What I realized that according to the USDA a product can be organic if it has five ingredients that are listed and known to be organic. Information from OrganicConsumers.Org states, "The word "organic" is not properly regulated on personal care products (example: toothpaste, shampoo, lotion, etc.) as it is on food products, *unless the product is certified by the USDA National Organic Program.*

Due to this lax regulation, many personal care products have the word "organic" in their brand name or otherwise on their product label, but, unless they are USDA certified, the main cleansing ingredients and preservatives are usually made with synthetic and petrochemical compounds.

Look for the USDA organic seal on personal care products that claim to be organic. Although there are multiple "organic" and "natural" standards, each with its own varying criteria, the USDA Organic Standards are the "gold standard" for personal care products.

If you want a product that is totally organic, look for the USDA organic seal. If it doesn't have the seal, read the ingredient labels to find out how many ingredients are truly organic and how many are synthetic." I believe that is a good food for thought especially in my marketing area which is home based. It's about a trust issue and informing my customers about homemade products by possibly introducing and educating them to the ingredients that are listed in a product from my garden where I grow about 70 percent of the herbs that are used.

The other percentage I actually obtain from a supplier that is certified organic.

Personally, I have used food coloring in the past because it was very attractive and a great marketing tool but after several months I decided to remove all dyes. Some products like soaps and shampoos are naturally dyed because of the plants particular coloring properties. Example, I make a Rose soap which is goat milk based but it has a nice rusk pink color because of the grounded rose hip powder that was used.

I realized while trying to market my products in a chain store known for its healthy and organic products that I would still have to add a synthetic harsh chemical ingredient to my products for undetermined shelf life. Fortunately, most homemade organic products can have a shelf life up to two years without harsh preservatives.

 My thoughts about my own products are that I would not probably have any products in any stores because of the compromise that I would have to make. That compromise is about money not the health of the consumer. Now not to say that all of my products are organic but I am definitely working towards that goal and customizing formulas as I too become aware of certain health restraints and issues.

There are a lot of products that have several different spin on organic and knowledge is the best resource for making appropriate decisions in regards to what you are willing to accept on your body and your head. Even words like herbal, organic, or natural really have no legal definition when it comes to cosmetic products and the word "Botanical" is defined as relating to plants or plant life. These makeup products must contain plant oils or properties in order to bear the "botanical" label. Botanical cosmetics typically do not contain any artificial or man-made ingredients. According to the Cosmetic Industry Dictionary Botanical is defines as a component of a cosmetic or personal care product that originates from plants (herbs, roots, flowers, fruits, leaves or seeds). Specific ingredients derived from biological sources are classified based on their chemical structure and how they are isolated from plants.

When purchasing your products remember you are the decision maker as a consumer and those that are providing a service for you are more concerned with mass marketing, great profits, and less expenses to give you what you think you need and at the end you are the one that is being double charged with your health.

Chapter 11   Hair Poetry

Who doesn't love poetry? I decided to throw in a few poems of my own reflecting on the time frame and hair attitudes that I was accustom to bringing awareness to the good, bad and ugly of natural hair.

Afro Queen

In your day after the ancients you reigned supreme

Your essence flowed and glowed

You were sought after and adored

You were bronzed and your body was radiant as if it had been poured.

You were laden with onyx, turquoise, diamond and gold

Your breastplate carved with stories untold

Your lips are full and body voluptuous with curves

As you sat upon your throne holding up the worlds

Men alike bowed down in your presence

And held your ankle gently in their hands

Kissed your feet that walked upon the desert sands

Stood before you patiently awaiting your audience

Admiring your radiance

No differences while they dreamt of mastering who you would be

But it's your hair Afro Queen which will define your history

Shine greatly with your natural mane and let the world see that you are finally free

A woman of your stature does not need a classification to BE

You just are an Afro Queen!

Hair Now & Then

When I was a child,

I knew nappy and kitchen before I knew real words

I burned from curling irons and straightening combs upon my head

I wore pink foams with plastic enclosures when I felt as if I was rich and used torn pieces of paper sack to roll my hair when I didn't have a stitch

When my hair was parted and made into plaits

I would be popped with a comb when I began to scratch

If I was patient enough excluding the tender head

I would sit for hours to have braids instead

My hair grease was Royal Crown and Murray's pomade

I would brush a hundred strokes to groom my mane

To disappear the ancestry of the family slave

To parade around with hair that was unnatural to be

But to get approval from those who despised me.

After thousands of dollars looking back as a grown woman

Switching from natural to relaxed and natural again

I see all that time and money we spend

On converting ourselves back to someone else's view and now that I am tired of being you

Finally accepting my hair and loving it as well

Now I see you wearing weave, extensions, dreads, and micro braids

I do not understand what you're trying to do

But please stop trying to be me and try to be You!

Hair Romance

Your hands are in my hair tugging gently to pull my head back to receive your many kisses

I smile at you with warm eyes because I know what you've been missing

You release the remainder of hair that is wrapped in a scarf tied upon my head

And shake out the curls that now lay upon the pillow of my bed

Your body is leaning over me strong cascading with abs that ripples across my bearing hips

You twist a strand of hair around your finger and brush it against my lips

Your breath is upon my cheeks slowly blowing the hair out of my face

I close my eyes waiting for your gentle embrace

You romance me from my head to my toes

The nature in us rose and rose

You breathe in my essence as I sighed much needed release

My hair mussed around my shoulders and your head resting upon my breast

I know that I am loved regardless if my hair is a mess

Naps versus Straight

Lil' nappy headed girl with pig tails and plaits

Where yo thank you be going wearing all of that

Hair so tight sticking close to your head

Lil' cuckabuds here there looking like you aint been fed

Why yo' hair don't grow all short and kinky

Look at mine's so sleek and slinky

See how my hair can blow in the wind

Your hair don't move it don't even bend

My momma presses my hair and dresses me too

I get my cloths hand me down from the neighborhood Jew

Did your mammy make yours from the Croaker Sacks?

Leftover from pulling cotton weighing on her back

See my hair is greased down and laying flat

Your niggah hair couldn't ever do that

I'm a grow up beautiful with pretty hair

And get me a black man that's light and fair

Yo man going be black and just as dark as you

"Cause you look like a jiggaboo

This nappy headed girl response to you

That times a changing with history

Its story will be told in a while

You still want be accepted because of your hair style

I choose to wear my hair natural versus you wearing yours straight

We are all ready divided and hair is not a debate

 Work on remaining true to your culture that's including your roots

So that one day we both can accept some truth

Brother

Deep brother that you are sharing your roots of masculinity

Proclaiming your throne from ancestral divinity

Those can tell the way you stride your Mandingo spirit

You cannot hide

Your strength is the coils that crown the glory of your head

I watched you walk by like Medusa with dreads

You spoke of the land where your ancestors dwelled

You reach into your being and your soul sprung forth like a well

The knowledge you shared was magnified by your appearance

When you spoke your peace there was no interference

A natural crown of glories and wisdom of brotherly stories

Brother you rein supreme your Nubian hair is a King

Kinky Hair

When I walk by I see you giving me the eye

If you're with your click of girls y'all mumble into each other's ears

But it's done in fear that I may hear

You think I am to black for you to understand

But, sometimes it's you that do not comprehend

I see you with your doe eyes, collagen lips and Botox smile

You act like you hate me but immolate me all the while

Your skinned is tan but not completely black

And you don't see how you're mentally attached

But, here you again want to play in my hair to satisfy some curiosity

Still behind my back you are mocking me

You want what I have but don't know how to get it

I see you with braids and now the dreads

Still trying to master the Afro on my head

I do not have to hide who I am inside

I accept who I am I do have pride

You keep on acting like you're afraid of me

But the only thing I see

Is you're trying to act just like me

Maybe one day we want give a damn about dark skin or natural hair

And that would be such a perfect world

But now I say to you buyer be ware

Here comes a sister with Kinky hair

Hair Journey

When I was a little girl my hair was picked, plucked, and plaited

Sometimes my hair was so tangled it became matted

It was then water brushed, pulled, and afro puffed

Sometimes I screamed at my hair in disgust

And then it became straightened with a hot comb

I didn't move in fear my forehead became a new home

A curling iron would clamp and roll on a parted section

I set in my chair like a spy avoiding detection

My hair was parted and put into corn rows

Afterwards I looked like a china man with a Negroid nose

Then came the beads that adorn my head making me feel pretty inside

I could swish my hair around mustering up my Black Pride

Then came the afro back on the scene like a mean machine

And you wore it with your fist held up high

Your fisted pick in your head tilting to the sky

Then I became conscious of society's thought

Not understanding fully what this had wrought

When I got my relaxer no more worries did I

I stuck by that box that was filled with toxic lye

I ran to the beauty shop to get that hair straight

Would go in early and come out late

And now after all the years from relaxer to weave

I finally had to accept and believe

It's okay to achieve the Natural look!!!

Chapter Twelve

Alex Story (a short excerpt)

Written by Alexandria Jones

Natural Hair: The "Root" of the Issue

"I wanted to straighten it." "I wanted to fit in." "I didn't like my hair." "I wanted it to be longer." "My mother made me." In a poll I conducted at my church, 15 African-American females ages 11-65 were asked, "Think back to the first time you straightened your hair.

Who or what made you do it?" The most common answer, by six people, turned out to be "My mother made me."

From the time most little African-American girls turn about 4 or 5, they are forced into getting a perm or getting their hair pressed. From barrettes to "red carpet ready", they are stripped of the chance to allow their own hair to naturally do what it does. A lot of the time, these little girls grow up to become women that look down on others of their own race that choose to embrace their own natural tresses.

It's not hard to understand why most people with naturally straight hair don't always see the beauty in the tightly coiled hair, given that they usually don't see it often or at all growing up.

What excuse do African-American's have? Is there something wrong with embracing "nappy hair?"

Why is it viewed as rebellious, rather than just being free to wear your own hair?

When the first slaves were brought to Jamestown in 1619, the norm of locks, plaits, and twists were essentially thrown out of the window. In 1865, slavery ended, but white people looked at black women who design their hair like white women as "well adjusted". These "good hair" styles became an essential for entering certain schools, churches, and social groups.
The Black Power movement, which aided in allowing blacks and whites to get a better understanding of each other, went on from 1960-1970.

Overall in 2011 chemical relaxer brands saw a significant decline in 2010, in Black women purchasing their products. Finally, in 2014, natural hair care products for Black women are a booming business.

In recent years, seeing that more and more people are "sticking to their roots" so to speak, the question of "Why do modern Black people themselves look down on people that embrace their own natural hair?" came to mind. I used to think that if anyone understood the mechanics of my hair, people of my race would. 'Tis not the case, In fact, I've seen that they are usually the main offenders, always asking if I cut my hair when I wear my usual afro. Some people have been so desensitized to the fact that they are basically changing themselves to fit in with straight-haired folks, that they don't see anything different as acceptable. Because they believe "good hair" is hair that a rat tail comb can go through without breaking, or that simply lays down straight. In fact, I see "good hair" as hair that is properly washed, moisturized, and has split ends clipped.

Good hair as it is called is really just healthy hair.

Some employers today will not employ people with locks or

Afros (whether Black or White) because it is "unprofessional" and "unkempt". Is it an act of rebellion to display your natural hair texture? That's not to say that kinky hair should look any old way, but why should people be turned down from a job because they choose to wear what is in the African-American culture's opinion suitable?

Sure, the corporate answer to this question is that there is a specific "image" expected to be upheld by the company. This "image" is sometimes what keeps employers from seeing the abilities of the person, due to their inability to see past the applicant's hairstyle.

On the flip side, I once got spring twists in my hair. During the amount of time that I had them, about 10% of compliments came from Black women. The remaining 90% came from one white guy my age, middle-aged white men and up. It was indeed fascinating.

This helped me remove the thought in my mind that white people simply did not like my natural hair. Sure, there are those that don't, but to see that there are those that can give a genuine compliment blew me away.

Some black people believe that to wear their own hair would mean that they are not as good as white people. Or just that it is easier to deal with when it is straightened. That is not to say that I believe pressing your hair is bad, just that one should not feel the need to change their outward appearance for someone or something else. Also, maybe our hair is actually very easy to deal with, and claims that it's easier when straightened are just an excuse. As someone who embraces my natural kinky hair texture, I know that it is very easy to maintain. All I have to do is wash, condition, rinse, moisturize, and pick. Three of these are done right in the shower and the remaining take only 5 minutes. What's really the issue?

In 2015, if you go outside sure you'll see racism, but there are so many people outside of the African-American race that are simply infatuated by the highly textured hair. This begs the question, "Is there something wrong with embracing 'kinky' hair?" I believe that the answer to this question is a solid no. I also believe that the solution to this problem is teaching young African-American children that their hair is beautiful. I asked my mother why she doesn't wear her own natural hair. Her response was, "My mama told me to as a child, so I had no choice. When I grew up it was all I knew. When I became an adult, natural hair was not embraced. I kept it straight so that I wouldn't stand out."

Until the age of about 10, a child's brain is like that of a sponge. This is an ample amount of time for a child to get the idea that their hair is sub-par. The root to the problem goes back to our African-American ancestors who changed their hair to be seen as acceptable to white women. The mindsets acquired during that time have been passed down through time, to this very day.

My mother began pressing my hair when I was about 2 or 3 years old. I continued to get my own hair pressed until the summer of 2014. Not being much of a hair person, I didn't know how to press my hair. Ever since the moment of enlightenment hit me, I have worn my afro ever since. I get my fair share of compliments, albeit, mainly from other people that wear their natural hair texture. Since then, my hair has actually grown, where in the past it used to break off a lot.

My goal isn't to convince people to stop flat ironing or perming their hair (though it can be damaging no matter what your hair texture is). I really want people to understand that kinky hair is not an abomination.

Perhaps one day, African-American's will see the beauty in their own hair, whether they don it or not. And in turn, other races will see that we won't stand down and respect us more for it, seeing that we respect ourselves. Regardless of our past as a world, we were and will always be pieces of a puzzle. The human doesn't make the hair, and the hair doesn't make the person. Our mindsets make us who we are.

The End

I thank you for reading my book and hope that it has favored you well.
Please take care of your hair it is part of your health.

Resources

Dr Ananya Mandal, MD *news-medical.net/health/Alopecia-What-is-Alopecia.aspx*

Dr Phoenix Austin, If You Love it, I Will Grow

Valerie Ann Worwood, the Complete Book of Essential Oils and Aromatherapy

www.Herbsinfo.com

www.blackgirllonghair.com

www.yahoo.com

www.livestrong.com

 www.ehow.com

http://www.wisegeek.com/what-is-mango-butter.htm

http://en.wikipedia.org/wiki/Shea_butter

http://www.theherbarie.com/Cupuacu-Butter.html

http://www.fruitsinfo.com/cupuacu-tropical-fruits.php

http://www.clutchmagonline.com/2011/03/10-butters-for-your-hair-and-skin/

http://www.naturalbeautyworkshop.com/my_weblog/2007/11/coffee-bean-but.html

http://www.ingredientstodiefor.com/item/Tucuma_Butter/1245

http://uniquelycurly.com/blog/2013/8/15/four-butters-other-than-shea-butter-your-hair-will-love

http://en.wikipedia.org/wiki/Macadamia

https://www.fromnaturewithlove.com/product.asp?product_id=BUTMURU

https://www.mountainroseherbs.com/products/kokum-butter/profile

http://www.livestrong.com/article/189783-the-benefits-of-hemp-oil-on-hair/

https://www.nenonatural.com/hair-blog/5-benefits-of-sweet-almond-oil-on-natural-hair

http://www.naturallycurly.com/curlreading/ingredients/just-peachy-peach-leaf-and-peach-kernel-oil-for-healthy-skin-and-hair/

http://allabouthealthyhair.blogspot.com/2013/07/what-is-best-carrier-and-essential-oil.html

http://www.curlynikki.com/2012/12/humectants-weather-and-hair-care-part-1.html

https://www.mountainroseherbs.com/products/kukui-nut-oil/profile

http://www.anniesremedy.com/herb_detail467.php

http://longing4length.com/what-does-the-grading-system-mean-for-hair-extensions.html

http://www.ebay.com/gds/Hair-Extension-Grades-A-to-AAAAA-Explained-/10000000177922838/g.html *http://www.feelgoodhairsupplies.com/article-What+is+your+human+hair+quality+grades%3F+What+is+the+best+sellers%3F-39.html*

http://blacknaps.org/know-your-hair-type/

http://blackgirllonghair.com/2012/03/natural-hair-type-guide-which-type-are-you/

http://www.goddessweaves.com/3a-grade-hair-vs-4a-5a-grade-hair-remy-vs-remi-knowledge-is-power

www.ingramcontent.com/pod-product-compliance
Lightning Source LLC
Chambersburg PA
CBHW060152290526
45789CB00003B/1007